Don't Be an Asshole Yoga Teacher

Don't Be an Asshole Yoga Teacher

A STUDIO OWNER'S PERSPECTIVE ON THE ETHICS OF TEACHING YOGA

Dr. Lisa Dana Mitchell

This book is dedicated to my teachers, my children, and every life experience that led me to become the person I am today. To my husband, for always pushing me and being my biggest fan: I am grateful.

Contents

Introduction

To be authentic yoga teachers, we must practice what we preach—in our thoughts, words, and actions. Generally, people who pursue teaching yoga do so because the practice has been beneficial and transformative to their own lives in some way. Hence, they want to share the many benefits with others. When we make the leap to teach yoga, we must have a conscious awareness that we are in a position of influence over the students. That is why it is so important to come from a place of compassion, honesty, and humility. Quite often, yoga students view their teachers as mentors, and they deserve to have a positive and trusting student-teacher relationship. As a yoga teacher, you have the opportunity to empower, encourage, and make a difference in the lives of so many, and this is truly a *gift* that we should all appreciate, respect, and be thankful for. I trust that this is the original and motivating intention of all individuals who teach yoga.

I have witnessed that once in the trenches of the yoga-teaching profession, however, many teachers cross the lines and let the game get dirty. Frankly, some teachers even start acting like, well, assholes. It is up to each of us as yoga teachers to implement the Yamas and Niyamas, not only to increase the professionalism of teaching yoga but to stay true to what yoga is all about.

I am co-owner of a family-owned chain of studios on the outskirts of Philadelphia. When we opened our doors in 2007, there were very few yoga studios around and, in particular, few to no heated Vinyasa studios in the area. In just a few short years, all of that changed—and changed drastically. People everywhere wanted yoga, and in all reality, that is a beautiful thing. A survey from the Sports and Fitness Industry Association stated that more than twenty-four million US adults practiced yoga in 2013, up from seventeen million in 2008. As these statistics show, more and more studios were opening their doors, and more and more yogis were signing up to become yoga teachers. In no way am I claiming that our business hasn't benefited from this growth in the yoga industry; however, the realities I have faced in running a yoga business have been challenging, in many ways shocking, and at times downright hurtful. I have learned many lessons along the way and hope to offer guidance in changing the current nature of this business, to be more aligned with the Yamas and Niyamas and to perhaps facilitate the business of yoga back into a more tranquil place, as I believe the sages intended.

Disclaimer: I completely acknowledge that there is an element of me being an asshole in writing this book. I clearly am not enlightened yet—maybe in the next lifetime! I am still excited to share my knowledge and my experience in the field of the yoga profession.

CHAPTER 1

The Ethical Rules of Yoga

Yoga has been mentioned in a variety of ancient texts, some dating back more than five thousand years. Such texts include the Vedas, Upanishads, and the Bhagavad Gita, to name a few. The credit for putting together a cohesive philosophy of yoga, however, goes to the sage Patanjali in the Yoga Sutras. In this spiritual text, Patanjali provided the very essence of the teachings of yoga in a highly systematic and somewhat scientific interpretation. The book is a set of 196 short, terse aphorisms or threads (sutras) that were intended to be read with repetition to the point of memorization.

Patanjali's Yoga Sutras has become an enormously influential work that is just as relevant for yoga philosophy and practice today as it was when it was written many years ago. The *sattvic* (pure) state of the yogi is described in great detail in the Yoga Sutras of Patanjali, which is a fundamental text on the attainment of yoga in your thoughts, words, and actions. The Yoga Sutras provide an outline of the specifics of behavior or habits that are present in the pure nature of a yogi and, for our purposes, the nature of a yoga teacher. It is also in the Yoga Sutras that Patanjali defines the first and second limbs of the Eightfold Path (Ashtanga Yoga), Yama and Niyama, which will be the primary focus of this book.

The Yamas and Niyamas are descriptions of how we are when we are living in union or yoga: connected, connected to our true self, and connected to all sentient beings. Rather than being just a list of do's and don'ts, the Yamas and Niyamas remind us that our fundamental nature is peaceful, compassionate, generous, and honest.

If you are presently a yoga teacher, you are hopefully already familiar with the other six limbs of Ashtanga Yoga. Still important to mention are Asana (physical postures), Pranayama (breath work), Pratyahara (withdrawal of the senses), Dharana (focus or concentration), Dhyana (meditation), and Samadhi (bliss state, or union with the Divine).

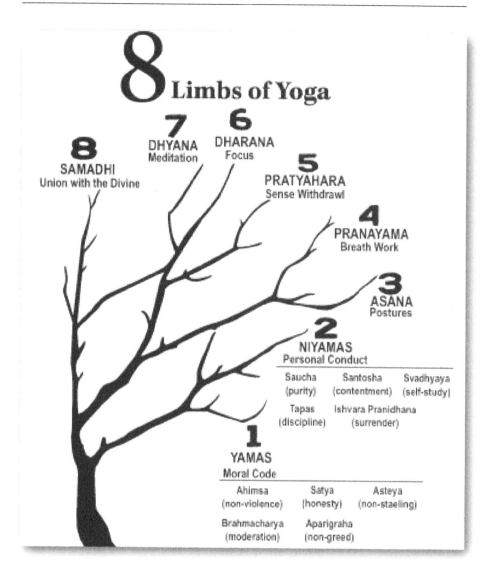

Let's start by focusing on the Yamas, as all other limbs build upon this one. The Yamas consists of characteristics essential to living a life on the path of freedom from suffering. The Yamas are concerned mostly with our outward experience and how we relate to others. Like any moral code you may have been taught as a youngster, the Yamas are restraints or things *not* to do. Yama is an essential part of the ethical code to living a yogic lifestyle. Hence, that is why I feel the Yamas are so critical, yet so easily forgotten in the process of teaching yoga.

As a supplemental way to absorb the ideas presented in this book, in each chapter I have included a yoga pose, a mudra, a mantra, and a journal prompt(s) to further incorporate each Yama and Niyama into your life and practice.

In the yoga practice, mudras are positions of the hands that have some kind of influence on the energies of the body. Usually, the hands and fingers are held in a particular position, but the whole body may be part of the mudra, as well. To most effectively use a mudra, hold the shape for at least a couple minutes. You will have an even more powerful effect with the mudra if you hold the finger-positions with both hands simultaneously.

When you select a word or series of words to repeat in the form of a mantra, you are affirming it's meaning and allowing the meaning to seep into your subcon-scious. Mantras, or sacred utterances, are most useful when done with repetition. The beauty of a mantra is that it can help to change your negative habits, thoughts and patterns into more positive habits, thoughts and patterns of behavior.

Lastly, journaling can be a highly meditative exercise as it has a profound effect on centering and grounding by bringing an added awareness to your experiences. It is also a valuable method to notice your strengths and weakness as you move forward in the path of yoga and yoga teaching.

I encourage you to use these supplemental activities as part of your practice and teaching, in an effort to feel more connected with your self, and inevitably connected to the students in your classes. Feel free to call on these supplemental activities when you feel a lack of a particular Yama or Niyama in your life, or if you ever question if your actions are on the realm of being an asshole or not.

CHAPTER 2

Ahimsa

Non-harming

True Ahimsa should mean a complete freedom from ill-will and anger and hate and an overflowing love for all.

—M. K. Gandhi

Negative thoughts give rise to violence...they are caused by greed, anger or delusion...Through introspection comes the end of pain and ignorance.

—Patanjali, Yoga Sutras

Non-violence leads to the highest ethics, which is the goal of all evolution. Until we stop harming all other living beings, we are still savages.

—Thomas A. Edison

himsa is usually translated as nonviolence, but this idea goes far and beyond the limited thought of not killing others, particularly in your role as a yoga teacher. Extending this compassion to all living creatures is dependent on our understanding and acknowledgment of the underlying union of all beings, with the scope of understanding way beyond just our friends, family, and pets. When we begin to recognize that the rivers of the earth are no different from the blood flowing through our own veins, it becomes very natural to extend compassion without any sense of doubt or restraint. Coinciding with the realization of oneness is the increasing difficulty of remaining indifferent to the problems and injustices of the world. You may notice a sense of hesitation in tossing trash onto the ground or cutting down a living tree simply because Ahimsa teaches that such acts would be an act of violence toward yourself, as well.

If you are a yoga teacher considering Ahimsa, it's helpful to ask yourself if your thoughts and actions are fostering the growth and well-being of all things. I firmly believe that for a yoga teacher, Ahimsa has many valuable components to consider.

What Does a Yogi Eat?

There is a mind-set and movement in yoga that suggests the quickest way to enlightenment is to put oneself in another's place and to see the oneness in all creatures. Through the practice of yoga, we gain a greater realization of the connectedness and union of all beings, and we strive to live in a harmonious fashion. This belief system endorses the idea that one of the best ways to put Ahimsa into practice is to cease eating the flesh of our animals and practice a vegetarian or vegan diet. Some feel strongly that yogis and yoga instructors in particular should not eat food that shares a connection with the pain or discomfort of other beings. The idea that a yogi should practice a vegetarian diet is one that is often in debate in the yoga community, but the idea suggests that eating animals is uncivilized and unethical.

In yoga classes across the globe, we hear the mantra "Lokah Samastah Sukhino Bhavantu," which translates to something akin to "May all beings be happy and free from suffering, and may my thoughts, words, and actions somehow contribute to that happiness and freedom." The argument for vegetarianism or veganism in the yoga community comes with the realization that the animals that we eat are often tortured and, obviously, killed. Therefore, when we eat animal meat and dairy, we are contributing to violence and harm to the animals.

As yogis, we want to create the least amount of negative karma as possible by doing the least amount of harm to others as we can—not to mention that raising animals for food creates more greenhouse gases than *all* the transportation (cars, trucks, trains, planes, ships) systems in the world. Raising animals for food causes more water pollution than any other industry. More than half the water consumed in the United States is used to raise animals for food. Forty-five percent of the total landmass of the United States is used to raise animals for food. An acre of forestland is destroyed every eight seconds to create more farms to confine animals raised for food. In the United States, more than 80 percent of corn crops and 95 percent of oats are fed to animals that are raised for food. Most of these crops are genetically manipulated and laced with pesticides. Wow!

So that is a lot to think about when we truly consider embracing Ahimsa more fully in our lives—something to consider before we post that filet mignon topped with blue cheese from dinner on our yoga Instagram accounts. Yum?

Physical Assists

As yoga teachers, an important consideration is to clarify when and why one might assist a student with physical adjustments. Yoga teacher training, combined with consistent personal practice and continued education in your craft, will sharpen your eye to really *see* your students and determine when a physical assist can inform a student on safer or more energetically aligned Asana, or physical postures. Assists can be useful in providing alternate ways to experience a pose. Physical assists can provide encouragement to your students, and sometimes they just feel downright "juicy" and "delicious," providing a deeper stretch, massage of muscles, and an amazing "aaaah" feeling.

When considering Ahimsa, however, it is OK to *not* touch people if you aren't 100 percent sure of what to do. Oftentimes, new teachers are so enthusiastic about teaching that they engage in physical adjustments and assists that can give the effect opposite of the intention. Think "eeeek" instead of "aaaah!" You may feel that the students aren't doing the pose "right" and they need a correction. You must realize as a yoga teacher that everybody and *every body* has a different experience on the mat while in the postures. We must take into account not just the yoga experience but, more importantly, *life* experience that people bring with them to the practice. A woman who recently had a baby may have a unique experience being postpartum; a person who was a serious athlete in college will also have a distinct experience in the postures based on the body's memory of the sport. We must also consider past trauma or abuse as well as injury and medical conditions when considering touch.

Oftentimes in teacher training, I suggest that physical assists should be done primarily on students you know, whose practice you are familiar with. That way there is a better understanding of how a particular body can be approached most safely and effectively.

Another useful strategy is to simply ask about any injuries or concerns that a teacher should be aware of and ask whether physical touch is a preferred method of learning for the student. If you choose the method of asking before class begins, please be mindful and do so with a level of confidentiality. You can have students wave a hand while the class is in child's pose, or you can simply be available before the class begins to meet and greet new practitioners, giving them the opportunity to share any issues or concerns they may be having that day. Some studios are even going as far as using a stone or some other symbol that the students can place in front of their mats if assists are OK for them. Calling people out to state traumas and injuries to a large group of people can be an asshole move that undoubtedly causes shame and embarrassment. The "calling-out method" of gaining this valuable information definitely should be avoided.

I cannot reiterate enough that we must make decisions based on Ahimsa when considering physical touch. If you wish to practice an exciting new assist that you just learned at a workshop or perhaps a juicy assist you were lucky enough to experience in your own body, I would suggest practicing with a peer (fellow yoga teacher) first before using students and paying customers as your guinea pigs. By practicing with a fellow teacher, you can receive valuable and informed feedback that can allow you the opportunity to refine your touch for your students.

I also acknowledge that not all teacher trainings place a strong emphasis on physical assists; some focus attention more on verbal cues. If you are not trained or confident in physical assists in your role as a teacher, then find a continuing education workshop or a teacher who can oversee you. It is the only way to ensure that yoga teachers are being guided through the lens of doing the least amount of potential harm to the students. Start small, working on mastering one particular assist at a time, building your repertoire slowly and effectively. Remember that the yoga practice is a practice of process, not attainment. Same for teaching! Enjoy the uniqueness, beauty, and oneness of all who step foot into your class. Strive to have the students feel freer in their bodies and in their breaths, as that is the highest form of yoga you can offer.

Verbal Language

As yoga teachers, we need to be mindful not only of physical assists that may cause harm if not done properly but also of the language we use to teach. We must refrain from using words that are condescending toward our students or that may create a sense of negative self-worth.

For example, instead of saying, "If you're not flexible, bend your knees," we can simply say, "Bend your knees if it feels right," or, "If it's available, straighten the legs." Our goal on the path of teaching yoga is one of empowerment and strength. We want our students to realize their potential, not be told that they are inflexible, not strong enough, or too big or too small to benefit from a posture. So, with Ahimsa, let's move beyond the obvious of physical harm and become more aware of the words we use when we teach and the potential effect these words have on others.

There are a few incidences that come to my mind when I reflect on our studio and past teachers who have used words that harmed the recipient. One student was extremely hurt by a teacher who exclaimed in the middle of an open class, "I have never seen the pose done like *that* before!" Of course, the student felt it necessary to share with me how hurtful her tone and words were and how it essentially ruined the practice for her that day. When I shared this feedback with the teacher, she claimed she was not even aware of how her words were perceived. I encourage you all to be aware and conscious at all times of your words when you are in the role of teacher...and really as just an individual in this world, throughout all of your interactions.

Another instance that comes to mind involved a female student who would wear layers of clothing, despite the "hot yoga" temperatures. A teacher whose class she frequented often would make occasional comments to her like, "Wow, aren't you hot?" or, "Oh my, those are a lot of clothes for hot yoga."

Finally, the student broke down and told her quite boldly that she suffered from body-image dysphoria and was just not feeling good about how she looked. That was why she would layer and not show any skin in class, despite the hot temperatures. She also expressed how the teacher's comments on her clothing and outfits for class were so inappropriate, judgmental, and downright rude.

Reality check for sure! As yoga teachers, we must have the awareness that all students come to the mat for their own unique and personal reasons. We are not to judge but rather to be open and compassionate vessels who provide the space for the practice to unfold for all individuals at their own pace and in their own special way.

I find it a good habit to forgive yourself for any incidences where you weren't as compassionate as you could have been. Recognize that you are perfectly imperfect and that every moment is an opportunity to strive to do better. Forgiving yourself will strengthen your capacity to love the full spectrum of who you are so that you can more readily and easily extend love to all others.

Let's Dig Deeper

Pose associated with Ahimsa: Virabhadrasana (Warrior I Pose)

From Downward Facing Dog, step your right foot to your right hand. Lower your back heel at a 30-45 degree angle and root through both feet as you lift the upper body away from the right leg. Stack the shoulders over the hips and gaze forward. Warrior I is considered a closed hip posture, so try to align your hips and torso to face forward. Repeat on left side.

Mudra associated with Ahimsa: Padma Lotus

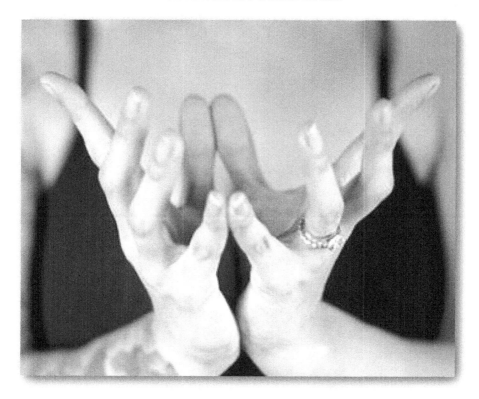

Bring your hands together at your heart with fingers apart, in the gesture of Padma (Lotus) Mudra. Draw inspiration from the innocence and determination of the lotus flower floating above the muddy waters of fear, desire and attachment. It is often such emotions that cause us to lash out in anger at ourselves and/or others.

Mantra: *Lokah samastah sukhino bhavantu*

Chant *Lokah samastah sukhino bhavantu* ("May all beings everywhere be happy and free from suffering") for three rounds.

When you are in pain -physical or emotional- describe at least three of the kindest thing you can do for yourself?

When I am in physical pain, I may need to focus on getting better sleep.
I also could take a warm shower or use soothing balm to alleviate my painful areas. I can pray about it & I also could do Yin yoga. massage.

If I am in emotional pain, I usually need to have some quiet space, or talk to a family member or friend. I also pray when I am in emotional pain & journal my prayers.

When you see someone else in physical or emotional pain, describe three kind things you can do for them.

LISTEN
HUG
SEE IF THEY WANT COMPANY / HELP
OFFER TO PRAY
~ SEND BOOK to Emma

CHAPTER 3

Satya

COMMITMENT TO HONESTY

The truths are easy to understand once they are discovered. The point is to discover them.

—Galileo Galilei

In a controversy the instant we feel anger we have already ceased striving for the truth, and have begun striving for ourselves.

—Buddha

As truthfulness (satya) is achieved, the fruits of actions naturally result according to the will of the Yogi.

—Yoga Sutra 2.36

This Yama is based on the premise that honest communication and honest action form the bedrock of any healthy relationship. On the flip side, deliberate deception, exaggerations, and mistruths are the bedrock of harming others. This goes back to Ahimsa again, as every Yama really just builds upon that one. The most effective way you as a yoga teacher can develop Satya is to practice honest speech. This means that when you say something, be as confident as possible of its truth. If we were to follow Satya with such conviction, we might find that we often have way less to actually say.

When you begin to consider what you say, you may notice that a large part of everyday comments and conversations that you have are not based upon what is known to be true, but are based on imagination, assumptions, often-erroneous conclusions, and sometimes full-on exaggerations. Remember, the truth is rarely convenient. One way you can know you are living with Satya is that while the choices you make may not be easy, at the end of the day, you can feel at peace with yourself.

Remove the Gossip

Gossip is probably the worst form of miscommunication. In fact, even the yogic text Hatha Yoga Pradapika (1:15) states that "talkativeness" and "gossip" are destroyers of yoga and should be avoided. With so many teachers nowadays, there is inevitably a lot of competition: competition to be on the schedule, competition over Instagram followers, competition over class attendance; the list can go on and on. People want to be the next big thing, even in the peaceful and calming yoga community. Although some level of competition can be healthy, it can also breed fear and a sense of inadequacy. When people are living in fear or with a sense of lack, it naturally becomes harder to be compassionate. I've heard a lot of gossip, trash talking, and tales of slander come down the yoga grapevine via social media outlets and in studio talk. The gossip can range anywhere from yoga teachers bashing other yoga teachers or differing yoga traditions, the student bashing the mentor, the teachers bashing the studio owner, friends bad-mouthing former friends who have become enemies—there are so many ignorant excuses for hurtful gossip.

I can identify specific occurrences of slander and gossip, but I would rather speak on behalf of them all. Human beings are innately flawed, imperfect, and often unbalanced and confused. Life can be messy, difficult, and hard to navigate. At times it feels as if we are just faking it until we make it, and perhaps that is precisely what we are doing.

There is nothing more negative or un-yogi-like than a person who gossips. You can visualize the body language of a gossip and see that it is an unattractive image. Imagine facial expressions of disgust and judgment, eye rolling, arms crossed against the chest: not quite the epitome of a yogi. I personally prefer to surround myself with people who are positive and enthusiastic, with people who love life. The students who show up for class want that, too. They want people who have optimism and passion about the practice to influence them. In my opinion, passionate people have less time for gossiping because they are spending so much of their time trying to actually do something positive in the world. Surround yourself with people who let passion—not degradation and gossip—be their yoga superpower.

Human beings are equipped with fantastic memories. In fact, the storage capacity of the human brain is limitless. So in the event that you have been the gossiper, people are going to remember. Think of your success in the yoga profession as being only as strong as your network of trusted peers and students. The wider your reach of trust in the yoga community, the wider your impact on it. Sure, we are human, and I admit that I can get excited over some juicy gossip at times, too. We all make mistakes and slip back into negative habits. But you best believe that gossiping can be a simple habit to cut out of your life. Trust that the benefits of dropping the gossip will far exceed the momentary sense of being the center of the wrong attention.

When You Don't Know, You Don't Know

I find it proper teacher etiquette to stick around after teaching to answer questions, to accept feedback, to chitchat, and to mingle with the community whenever possible. In my years of teaching, I have had a myriad of questions from students...most questions being about chaturanga and downward-facing dog. Yet on occasion, you get the students asking questions about injuries, past or present, which can be very complicated and intricate to answer. You may even hear key anatomy terms like ACL, hip flexor, patella, and rotator cuff thrown around. You are likely to have some familiarity with these terms from the study of anatomy in your yoga teacher training. As yoga teachers, however, we are not medical doctors (unless you are). We must be willing to admit when we just don't know the answer to a question. It is crucial that we do not misrepresent our scope of knowledge. If a student approaches you after class with a question that you are not sure about, be honest, speak your truth, and admit that you don't know, if that is the case. Offer to investigate the question and have an answer for him or her at a future class if this is a consistent student. Perhaps refer him or her to someone who may know: a studio owner, a more experienced teacher, or even a medical professional. You will gain more respect with authenticity than in faking the funk. Yogis are often intuitive enough to notice when you are not living Satya anyway.

Be Real About Who Shows Up

Another aspect of Satya that we must face is being honest with who shows up to class. Oftentimes teachers, especially newer teachers, get very excited about creating flows and sequences that include arm balances, handstands, intricate transitions, and the like. Then they walk into the studio, and it is full of beginners.

You must plan ahead but be flexible enough to change on the spot based on the realities of the class. I recommend that you keep it simple and know options to build on if more intermediate or advanced practitioners show up. A class that has a strong foundation, that touches each body part in a safe and logical way, is often the most profound class for the students.

In business, there is an 80/20 rule, where 80 percent of sales are made by 20 percent of the consumers. This 80/20 rule also applies to many other facets of business, and I feel it is applicable as well in yoga teaching. You are not looking at the perspective of sales in this case, but you can use this equation to determine and gauge your teaching in the moment. For example, if 80 percent of the class is keeping up with your pace, then you are on the right track. There will always be those few (20 percent or so) that will be moving slower or faster than your cues, but if fewer than 80 percent can keep up, maybe you need to cue slower and vice versa.

Another example: if 80 percent of the class can accomplish the poses you are offering, you are again teaching with an awareness of who is actually in the room. There will always be those few (20 percent perhaps) that will go beyond the scope of your offerings and intensify the poses with alternate variations, and in that 20 percent will be those who need more intense modification. The 80/20 rule is a good gauge in yoga teaching and a sure way to adjust your teaching as needed in the moment.

We must also be comfortable, yet supportive, when being honest with students who are not moving through poses in the most beneficial way for them or who are practicing poses that are not appropriate for them at the time. If you see students struggling in a upward-facing bow (urdhva dhanurasana), for example, to a point that they are creating an unsafe circumstance in the body, you must be honest enough to approach them and offer an alternative—even if that means advising them to come out of the pose to take a more simplified version. It can be awkward, and it may even shatter the students' egos, but it is the best practice when keeping students safe and honest with themselves.

We should honor where the students are, suggest they honor where they are, too, and always reiterate that there is no rush in moving to more advanced poses. I often remind students that yoga is a lifelong practice, and if we are lucky, we can just try again tomorrow, and the tomorrow after that, and the tomorrow after that, and so forth. I always hope that the students will honor the teacher's guidance and realize that feedback and suggestions to scale back in a pose are in their best interest. Honesty always, my friends!

Be Real about You

As a teacher, you must be authentic, honest and have integrity. You must be *real*. Stop the yoga teacher persona and any pretending, and feel confident that others will be attracted to your true self. Your students will admire your being yourself, a bit vulnerable, and open to your own mistakes as well as accomplishments on this path of yoga. Only when you are honest about yourself will the students trust you enough to be their most authentic selves, too. When you are truthful about yourself, you will find easier longevity in your teaching. Who has the time and energy to "pretend" anyway?

With Satya, the off-the-mat you is just as important as the you on it. Make sure your social media outlets present a true version of yourself, not the idealized version you think students want you to be. It is always nice to post your most perfect pose, but your students will really appreciate the bloopers or the realness of what goes into mastering such aesthetic perfection. This also gives the honest reality that with practice, all really is coming.

Your Voice Matters

When we think of Satya as a way to speak your truth, it is important to address your voice (literally) as a yoga teacher. Take notice if you put on a yoga teacher voice when you teach or if you maintain your natural talking voice. Aside from inflection that occurs to set the tone of a sequence, I recommend the latter. Part of utilizing your most authentic voice is to do just that.

I also recommend cleaning up the language you use while you teach. Notice the areas where you add unnecessary words into your cues and rid those from your instruction. Words and phrases such as "um," "now go ahead…" and "now we are gonna…" are fillers that offer no help to your students and take up precious time. When you offer cues to the class, think "verb, body part, direction." For example: "Step your feet to the top of the mat" or, "Reach your arms overhead." Practice being concise, and you will notice the class can more effortlessly follow your cues. Teach as if you are giving directions to a ten-year-old. No, seriously.

All great writers and speakers know about the importance of editing. (I just cut and pasted a paragraph before I wrote this one.) Oftentimes, the shorter and simpler you keep your narratives, the better.

Have you ever experienced a teacher who goes on and on while you are holding a difficult pose? The teacher just keeps reiterating for you to "just relax, let it go, ignore the pain, *breathe into the pain…*"

And all you can think is, "Get me out of this pose!"

I have even been tempted to throw a yoga block or two at a teacher during such circumstances. Keep it short and sweet. Think about what you want to say, and evaluate if it is a necessary truth. Will your words add to the dialogue, or are you just nervously filling the silence? I have been guilty of this myself as a new teacher, feeling as if I needed to fill up every nook and cranny with words so I didn't have to really open myself or be vulnerable. Silence can be scary. But there are times when students need silence in order to practice control of their breaths as well as to practice the valuable control of their minds.

I attended training in Lancaster, Pennsylvania, years ago. I was already a yoga teacher, but I am always a proponent of furthering my training whenever possible. We participated in an activity where we did a "popcorn" yoga class, meaning we all took a turn teaching a segment of a class, building from where the person prior left off. We were instructed to call out feedback to our peers in the moment, so if someone needed to be louder, we could just call out, "Talk a little louder," and so forth.

So when it was my turn to teach, I was feeling super confident. Being a yoga teacher already, I felt very prepared to share every bit of knowledge I had about the Asanas. So there I went, cueing and cueing, sharing and describing every detail of each pose fully.

Finally one of the peers in my group screamed out violently, "Just stop talking!"

I was flabbergasted. I was hurt; I went into the bathroom of the studio with a lump in my throat, convinced that I was never coming to this training again. I was calling this woman every type of nasty swear word in my head. Yet this was probably some of the most pertinent feedback I ever received. Rather than trying to be impressive with unnecessary words, I now teach to what I see. I strive to speak only what needs to be said. It is so much more powerful to teach this way. I encourage you to give it a try!

Asking for Subs Much?

Another important aspect of Satya as a yoga instructor occurs around your dependability as a teacher. Consider when and why you call out or find coverage for your classes. Are you being honest when you say you can't make it in to teach and seek a sub, or are you choosing not to maintain your obligations? The students rely on us for so many reasons, and when we consistently call out, we are often disappointing them. Therefore, be honest; if teaching yoga is really what you want to be doing, show up! I cannot tell you how many times students will leave or express great disappointment when the regularly scheduled teacher calls out consistently or has a sub. It is true: people want to be in your presence, so honor that commitment as much as possible.

Let's Dig Deeper

Pose associated with Satya: Anjanayasana (Crescent lunge)

From Downward facing dog, step your right foot forward and lift your back heel so you are on the ball of your back foot. In this pose, all toes are pointing forward. Engage your lower belly and reach your arms over your head, or choose to take the hand mudra associated with this Yama. Stay for five full deep breathes. Repeat on the left side.

Mudra associated with Satya: Kali Mudra

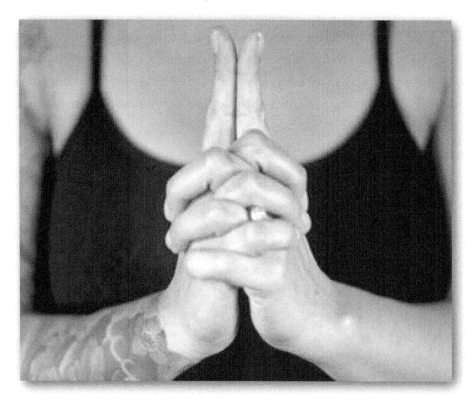

Bring the hands together with all fingers interlaced except your index fingers. This mudra is named after the fierce goddess Durga. Kali and Durga are manifestations of the goddess Mahadevi. Durga represents the empowerment that enables us to stand in our own truth. The index fingers represent the sword of Durga, who slays illusions, false understandings, and ignorance.

Mantra: *Sat nam*

Inhale to lift the hands overhead, and exhale to lower them to heart center. You can visualize your sword cutting through whatever causes you to be dishonest, insincere or inauthentic. Repeat this movement three times while chanting the mantra *Sat nam* ("My name is truth").

Write at least 10 words or phrases you need to hear.

I Love you

Good Job

You're doing great

Keep doing your best

I'm sorry

I forgive you

Let's do it together

You're the Best

Your hard work shows

I Know you can do it

If your body could talk it would say...   Honor me

There have been many years I have
taken it for granted.

Feed me better

Thank you for taking care of me.

Thank you for making wise choices

I like to be pushed / work hard

Love me for who I am.

Don't compare me to others.

CHAPTER 4

Asteya

NON-STEALING

Once you realize that the source of all solutions that you seek outside yourself is always present within you, asteya naturally happens.

—Yogi Amrit Desai

When nonstealing (asteya) is established, all jewels, or treasures present themselves, or are available to the Yogi.

—Yoga Sutra 2:37

The desire to possess and enjoy what another has, drives a person to do evil deeds. (It) includes not only taking what belongs to another without permission, but also using something for a different purpose to that intended, or beyond the time permitted by its owner.

—B. K. S. Iyengar

steya arises out of an expressed feeling of inadequacy or deprivation. It comes from a feeling of "not being good enough" and a doubt that we are able to manifest what we need by ourselves. This mind-set can lead to stealing in a variety of ways far beyond just physically taking something from someone else. We often waste our time hoping for some better life or envying the lives of others who appear to have the things we desire. When constantly looking outside ourselves for satisfaction, we are less able to appreciate the abundance that already exists *within* us. Yoga teaches us that what really matters is our health, the gifts that are present in all of us, and the joy and love we are able to give and receive from others. It becomes difficult to appreciate that we have hot running water when all we can think about is which hundred-dollar yoga pants to purchase next.

The practice of Asteya asks us to be careful not to take anything that has not been freely given. The paradox of practicing Asteya is that when we relate to others from the vantage point of abundance rather than from neediness, we find that others are more generous with us. Life's greatest treasures will begin to flow your way.

Stealing Time

Have you ever been to a yoga class that started fifteen minutes late or went over-time by twenty minutes? Well, this is 100 percent stealing the students' time! When we do not honor the times posted on a yoga schedule, we are taking advantage of the students and, in fact, stealing their time right from them. Understand that making it to a yoga class requires students to carve out a particular amount of time from their life to practice and taking more or giving less is just not fair. I had a yoga teacher go over a class by thirty minutes one time. I personally didn't have somewhere else to be that day, so it didn't result in my being late for the next thing on my schedule. In fact, I was really enjoying the class, so I didn't even notice that the class lasted longer than what was advertised, but when I walked outside after class, I had a parking ticket. The extra thirty minutes caused my meter to expire. Whomp, whomp—a yoga teacher fail in my opinion.

Also, notice your own presence as a teacher. If your mind is somewhere else and you are not in the moment when teaching, you are essentially stealing the students' time then, too. Maintain present moment awareness, and you will be able to give more fully to the class and students. Trust me, it becomes very obvious when the yoga teachers are checked out, distracted by their playlists, their personal lives, and the like There is a yoga teacher at our studio who is very honest when her personal life interferes with her teaching. She has the awareness to know when her thoughts have been pulled in another direction and never wants to create a disservice to the students. I completely admire this and am always open to letting her take the time she needs to feel more present to teach. This is a true example of how living in her truth (Satya) allows her to not steal from the students in her classes.

Stealing as We Know It

I assume it goes without saying that we should not be stealing from the studio's registers, refrigerator, or yoga supplies. Now that would definitely be an asshole thing to do. But I will go further to suggest you do not steal a studio's clients, either. Oftentimes the professional yoga teacher will teach at a variety of studios in the surrounding areas. In many cases, this is a necessary task, if a yoga teacher intends to create a functional living. However, teachers should not be soliciting a studio's clientele for non-studio-related yoga offerings. If a teacher intends to host yoga retreats or teacher trainings independent of the studio, and the studio already offers their own retreats and trainings, then this is a conflict of interest. I have many yoga studio owner cronies, and we can all agree that soliciting events at a studio without studio affiliation is a no-no. This is a poor and unhealthy analogy, but imagine advertising Burger King inside a McDonald's.

But the plot thickens. I have witnessed yoga teachers log in to online client information systems, get client names and e-mails, and seek out studio customers via social media platforms. I guess that is not soliciting *within* the studio—but hmmmm, ask yourself if you can rest easy after doing such a thing.

I will share a policy that a studio owner peer has suggested to combat this situation. When a yoga teacher hosts a retreat independent of a given studio, the studio shall receive a small portion of retreat profit from all attendees who are members of that particular studio. This way, there is no sneakiness involved, and the studio and the teachers will then promote the event cohesively, as a unit, together. This is a win-win for everyone, creating community versus separation, as well as opening up the offerings and the clientele on a larger scale. Not sure if this idea will ever come to fruition, but I would love for the conversation among studio owners and teachers to further develop.

A perception among studio owners is that many yoga teachers attempt to build their own personal yoga business off the backs of the hard work the studios have already set forth. Sometimes I say "whatever" and don't really care, but other times, when I really think about it, it just feels like an asshole way to be as a yoga teacher.

Learn to Share

The greatest gift of having knowledge is the ability to share this knowledge with others. In yoga, there is no "yours" or "mine." Let go of the thoughts that other teachers are stealing your sequences or ideas and make peace with a sharing of inspiration instead. Create a mentality built on abundance, and practice nonattachment. (We will get into non-attachment a bit later). It is a beautiful thing to take a class and be inspired to later share a flow, sequence, or quote that you experienced with another teacher. And imitation is a great expression of admiration. So even if a teacher "steals your sequence," the exciting thing about being a yoga teacher is that no one can be you! So even if someone were to use even your exact words, the experience will still never be the same as when you taught it. Honor the uniqueness of who you are as a teacher. Consider giving kudos to those who inspire you. Express your yoga teachings freely, without agenda or need for accolades for your offerings. Remember, the opposite of sharing is stealing.

"Your Students"

"Comparison is the thief of joy." That quote resonated with me after a handstand workshop with Kathryn Budig, although the original quote was from Eleanor Roosevelt. (See, I just gave an example of giving kudos to someone who inspired me.) In the business of yoga, stop comparing yourself to other teachers. It is always a nice reminder that no student is "yours." Stop using phrases like "my students, my following," or, "I taught them that." When students transform or improve, *they* should get the credit for it. Quiet the ego that fools you into thinking that you are more important than this sacred and transformative practice of yoga.

I have found even the most packed of classes on a schedule have a variety of reasons for being busy. Yes, an experienced and/or passionate teacher does help. One must consider convenience of the customer, however, as a major player in determining which classes are most attended. I have had senior teachers give up a time slot, and although they would be missed, a large majority of the students still show up to that class despite the teacher, simply because that particular day, time, and location works for them. Remind yourself that it's not always about you. Otherwise, you'll find yourself trying to hold on to "your" students, with an attachment to attendance that inadvertently steals the joy out of your own teaching.

Let's Dig Deeper

Pose associated with Asteya: Virabhadrasana III (Warrior III)

From Crescent Lunge, place your hands at your heart and shift your weight forward. Lift your back leg until it parallels the earth, initiating movement from the inner thigh to maintain your hips in a level position. You can imagine the body as a shape of a capital T in this asana. Warrior III reminds us to seek balance in all aspects of life.

Mudra: Hasta (Hand) Mudra

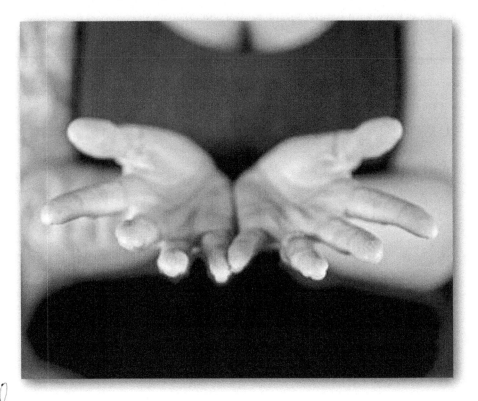

Hasta Mudra is a heart opening mudra, and represents a gesture of both giving and receiving. Reach your arms out and radiate your upturned palms, releasing the fear and illusion of not having enough.

Mantra: *Om shrim lakshmiyei namaha*

Summon the power of Lakshmi, the goddess of light and abundance, by chanting *Om shrim lakshmiyei namaha*. Only when you feel you have all that you need, you won't feel the need to take anything from anyone else.

Identify what is *enough* for you?

_____
_____
_____
_____
_____
_____
_____
_____
_____
_____
_____
_____
_____
_____
_____
_____
_____
_____
_____
_____
_____
_____
_____
_____
_____
_____
_____
_____

Identify three ways that you allow others to steal your valuable time?

Participating in activities
I don't really want to. —
Obligation

Hanging out w people I don't want to

Responding to texts I don't have time
or energy for

CHAPTER 5

Brahmacharya

MODERATION, ABSTINENCE

Everything in Moderation, including moderation.

—Julia Child

Love begets courage, moderation creates abundance and humility generates power.

—B. K. S. Iyengar

Desires never fulfill anyone. Buddha has said it is not the nature of desire to be fulfilled. Fulfillment comes only by lack of desire.

—Osho

Of all the Yamas, Brahmacharya might be the least understood and the most feared by Western yogis. Commonly translated as "celibacy," this principle creates turmoil in the minds of those who interpret Brahmacharya as a required act of sexual suppression. Practically all spiritual and religious traditions have wrestled with the dilemma of how to use sexual energy wisely. Practicing Brahmacharya means that we use our sexual energy to regenerate our connection to our spiritual self. It also means that we don't use this energy in a wasteful way or in any way that might harm others. There goes that Ahimsa again.

It may be easier to understand Brahmacharya if we remove the sexual connotation and look at it more on an energetic level. The word *Brahmacharya* actually translates as "behavior that leads to Brahman." Brahman is thought of as "the creator" in Hinduism, so what we're basically talking about here is behavior that leads us toward "the divine" or "higher power." When we regard Brahmacharya as the "right use of energy," it allows us to consider how we actually direct our energy, as both yoga teachers and individuals. Brahmacharya also evokes directing our energy away from external desires, from those pleasures that seem great at the time but are ultimately short-lived and momentary. Brahmacharya suggests that we instead strive to find peace and happiness within ourselves, accentuating yoga as an inward practice.

Student/Teacher Relationships

As a yoga teacher, it is critical to observe student-teacher relationships and have firm boundaries in relations with students. In other words, don't sleep with your students. If you have an overpowering connection to a student that cannot be resisted, then by all means, pursue. Just do not have that person be your student in a yoga studio or place of employment anymore.

In addition, any flirtatious chitchat should not be done within a studio of employment. I would advise having such conversations in an alternate location, to maintain a sense of professionalism in the studio space. I think having the opportunity for couples to practice together can be a beautiful thing; having your mats side-by-side and holding hands in shavasana can be so romantic. In fact, some of my favorite dates with my husband are yoga dates. The dynamic of someone in your class who was once your student but now is your lover, however, can lead to a myriad of problems.

As a studio owner, I see that when teachers date students (against my moral advice), it can create problems for the business as a whole. Say your significant other comes to your class, and you just can't help but give him or her a little extra attention. The students then notice that most of your attention is clearly not on them. We all know that a relationship can fog our best judgment, especially in the workplace. Or imagine when you break up. Is it fair that the studio has now just lost a consumer because of your indiscretions with students?

Or perhaps the heartbroken ex wants to retaliate and continues to take your classes, despite you not wanting him or her there. Now you have to navigate teaching with the emotional attachment or distraction that exists in the class. As you can see, it can get tricky for the overall vibe of the studio, as well as in your own teaching.

In the field of psychotherapy, there are very strict rules and regulations around befriending clients or having romantic relationships with them. According to recent regulation, a therapist can befriend a client one full year after termination of therapy and must wait two full years after terminating a therapeutic relationship to become romantically involved with the client. At this present time, there are no clear ethical standards set for yoga teachers. Standards may differ from one individual situation to the next, but I find that with the subtle nature of yoga teaching and with the emotional vulnerability of students, we must at least take into consideration the guidelines as addressed by the regulations of psychotherapy.

There is no doubt that male teachers are generally faced with different challenges than female yoga teachers. This is partly due to the fact that the majority of participants in a public class tend to be female. They also need to be mindful about how they give adjustments, as well as the intention behind the assist, as we mentioned in the chapter on Ahimsa and will touch on again in a moment. Great advice from a male (married) yoga teacher peer that I often share is that if he feels that a student has an intimate intention in attending his classes, he refrains from assisting that individual at all. That way, no obscure lines get crossed, and no mixed signals get sent. Not bad advice, in my opinion.

In a quick Google search, you can find horror stories of yoga teachers and perceived "gurus" who have overstepped boundaries with students and been accused of rape, economic manipulation, sexual assault, and cultlike practices that have violated students' sense of self and overall well-being (but I will not be the one to gossip). Such behavior is the polar opposite of what we should strive for as yoga teachers. Such abuse of power has no doubt created irreversible damage to the students involved, whose only fault was that they admired the teachers in such a way that they were unwillingly manipulated and controlled. This has also caused the demise of several schools of yoga, as well as student disassociation with particular teachers and teaching styles in the yoga world on a massive level.

Having a standard of neutrality in student/teacher relationships should be a goal. Yet, there are many yoga teachers who successfully befriend their students and socialize with them outside the studio without a negative outcome. I have witnessed this type of friendship be very healing for both the student and the teacher. In fact, Krishnamacharya (deemed the father of modern yoga) said that the best kind of teacher *is* actually a good friend. I will remind you, however, that teachers need to remain clear about the nature of the relationship. If there is an equal peer-to-peer relationship, healthy friendships between the student and teacher are definitely possible. Being a yoga teacher requires an intense amount of self-reflection and honesty in terms of boundaries. Consider these three things when expanding boundaries with your students:

1. What is the student's motivation?
2. What is your motivation?
3. What is in the best interest of the student?

When taking into consideration these three factors, you find it easier to realize any ulterior motives that may interfere with a healthy friendship dynamic in your role as a teacher.

Where Is Your Gaze?

We must also be mindful of how we are perceived as teachers. Tune in to how you dress and how you touch your students. Do not build a reputation of being the seductive or perverted yoga teacher! Even though I fully believe we are all divine souls and spiritual beings, I do feel that some assists can be sketchy when performed on the opposite sex. There are amazing down-dog assists, for example, that I just would not perform on a female student if I were a heterosexual male teacher—like placing my hands between a student's legs to pull the thigh bones back. Again, a juicy assist, but it also can be a precarious hand placement on a woman.

We must also be mindful of where our gaze is when we touch students. There is no doubt that we can get in close: buttocks in our faces, breasts pressed against us, see-through pants in the room, you name it. We see it all as yoga teachers. We must be constantly aware of where our eyes are looking.

True story: One male teacher was assisting an intermediate female student in a handstand. A fairly common assist consists of placing a fist between a student's thighs and giving a verbal cue to squeeze the inner thighs strongly against the fist. In this particular instance, the student squeezing the fist in handstand was fine with the assist. Another practitioner observing the handstand and physical adjustment, however, felt it was inappropriate, based on the way the teacher was looking at said student.

Dancing Drunk on a Bar

When you are a yoga teacher, students in your classes look up to you. They hold you in high esteem and admire that you have a skill set and understanding of yoga deeper than their scopes of the topic. They may also look to you as an icon of health and wellness in many cases. It is sometimes difficult for people to realize how people view you when you become a yoga teacher, but this preconception is often very true.

I recommend, when out in public, practicing moderation with alcohol and (of course) illegal substances. The joke that we have in teacher training is, "By all means, still enjoy yourself, but don't be the drunk person dancing on the bar!" Brahmacharya teaches us that we must use moderation in activities that waste our energy and take us further from being in control of our senses.

In modern yoga of the Western world, there is definitely a trend of thinking like, "Sometimes I drink green juice, and sometimes I take tequila shots. It's called moderation." Yes, in some capacity that is moderation. As a yoga teacher, however, I suggest abandoning the old habits that stand in the way of your truest self, and if those involve excessive drinking, then so be it. Besides, who wants to teach the 6:00 a.m. yoga class with a hangover?

I assure you that when you envelop yourself in the yoga practice and decide to live with Yamas and Niyamas as a manifesto, you will naturally choose to have other means of socializing, and you may even notice that your friendships evolve and you surround yourself with people who have similar interests. It is true that like attracts like. For some, what I am saying may not be easy. Being a yoga teacher isn't easy, but we have chosen (or perhaps been chosen) to live that path, right?

Let's Dig Deeper

Pose associated with Bramacharya: Balasana (Child's Pose)

Come onto your knees with your toes touching, and your seat resting over your heels. Relax your belly on your thighs. The restorative and inward nature of this pose fosters the parasympathetic nervous system to facilitate relaxation and rejuvenation.

Mudra: Prana Mudra

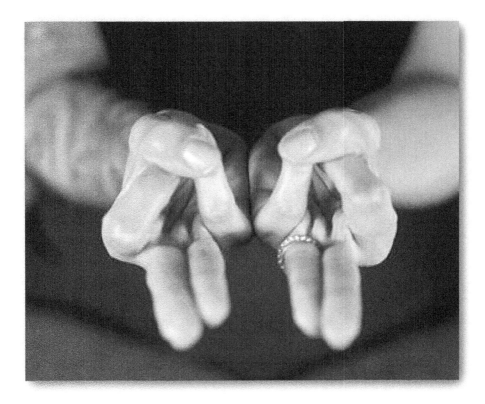

Extend your arms forward and bring your thumb, ring, and pinky fingers on each hand to touch, while lengthening the index and middle fingers. This gesture of Prana Mudra elicits the vitality that resides within our prana, or life force.

Mantra: *Om somaye namaha*

Chanting the mantra *Om somaye namaha* calls upon the rejuvenating nectar (soma) that drips from the moon in Hindu mythology. This nectar is intended to wash away the stressors of life that leave you feeling depleted and worn down.

Dear Past Me . . .

Dear Future Me . . .

_____

_____

_____

_____

_____

_____

_____

_____

_____

_____

_____

_____

_____

_____

_____

_____

_____

_____

_____

_____

_____

_____

_____

_____

_____

CHAPTER 6

Aparigraha

NON-ATTACHMENT, NON-GREED

Travel Light, Live light, Spread the light, Be the light.

—Yogi Bhajan

Why court the impossible? Why undertake to solve a puzzle that cannot be solved? Think about it carefully. How else will you learn to drop your attachment to the fruits of your actions? When hope for success remains, attachment to the results will persist. When you pit yourself against the impossible, Nonattachment to the results is your reward. This is how you'll know your dharma and move mountains to execute it.

—David Garrigues

Dare to live by letting go.

—Tom Althouse

parigraha is an important Yama that teaches us to take only what we need, keep only what serves us in the moment, and let go when the time is right. As you may have already discovered, when we try to hold on too tightly to anything, whether it be our relationships or our material items, the grasping often leads to the demolition of those very things we most covet and crave. Our best security lies in detaching from strong feelings of jealousy so we can take down the walls that block our own growth as individuals. Only when we let go of desire and attachment can we be vessels of growth and resilience.

Aparigraha is one of the central teachings in the yogic text the Bhagavad Gita. Krishna shares perhaps one of the most important teachings of all: "A gift is pure when it is given from the heart to the right person at the right time and at the right place, and when we expect nothing in return." What Krishna is essentially saying is that we should never concern ourselves with the outcome of a situation or action. We should concern ourselves only with what we are doing and, more specifically, the intention behind it. Let go of worrying about recognition of your actions, stop wondering if you are "good enough," and trust that you have been called to share your gifts by something far grander than yourself. This is how you can pursue your *dharma* or duty of teaching yoga as it aligns with Aparigraha or nonattachment. Have faith that you have been called to teach, that you have a gift to share. Otherwise, why would you be teaching?

Getting on the Schedule

Wow, how exciting it is to get a spot on the schedule at the studio you trained with or even a studio you enjoy practicing at. (Side note: I always recommend teaching at studios where you actually like to attend classes, so that your vision, vibe, and teaching style can be in alignment.)

Fresh out of teacher training, however, you may have to be OK with sub-bing. Open yourself up to being on the sub list, as this is a great first step to getting a permanent position. I have seen firsthand how competitiveness can occur when teachers are fresh out of training and everyone wants a spot on the schedule. I have witnessed friendships dissipate, with a lot of he said/she said occurring within the studio. (There goes that gossip again.) This is a clear example of not only greed and attachment, but also jealousy that breeds from desire and wanting. The Yoga Sutras teach us to replace our negative thoughts with more positive ones, so when those feelings of jealousy or resentment occur around who is teaching where, and the like, it is a perfect opportunity to put such yogic principles into action. Instead, be happy for your peer, and trust that as long as your intentions are pure, your opportunity will come. Keep expressing your interest in teaching, keep practicing, remain a member of the community, and you will remain in the mix when classes open up. You must also take into account that only when a studio is new or expanding will there be many teaching spots to fill. If such an expansion is not happening, a studio will have an opening only if a teacher leaves or the studio decides to add additional classes. So please, be patient.

As a new teacher, you may be offered a time on the schedule that is not a prime-time teaching spot. Think 5:45 a.m., for example. If you are offered a non-preferred time spot and it is feasible for your schedule, by all means, take it. Do not hold out for the busiest class times on a schedule, as studio owners have to be mindful of who teaches when. They may prefer more experienced teachers during the busier classes. Packed classes require a more adept knowledge of teaching to a larger and broader group of yogis; however, the hypothetical 5:45 a.m. class will give you the opportunity to gain that valuable experience, to get a busier time slot down the road.

If a studio has an unoccupied time on the schedule, propose it to the studio owner and express your interest in getting the class started. I had a teacher shoot me an e-mail proposing an 8:00 a.m. class time. She stated reasons why she thought that could be a valuable addition to the schedule and stated she was fine with it being a "trial" class for three months to see if it could create a client base. Her initiative and proposal were enough for me to say, "Sure, let's give it a go." I appreciate a teacher's initiative and will likely go with an idea if I can see and feel the teacher's passion.

Don't Be Greedy

Those of us who have gone through yoga teacher training contemplate quitting our day jobs to teach yoga full-time. Whether the thought is acted on or not, it is often considered. Many of us, in fact, do quit our jobs and pursue full-time yoga teaching. Don't quit your day job so fast, however. Know that to live without greed as a yoga teacher, you must realize your worth in relation to your experience and expertise. I would recommend offering free or cheap privates to friends and family for quite some time, to gain valuable experience, before you start charging an overpriced $150 per hour when you're fresh out of teacher training. In the practice of yoga, as in the practice of teaching, we cannot rush the process. When we are authentic in our way of being as teachers, abundance will naturally come.

If money becomes the motivation for teaching yoga, you will likely not find success. Remember, we are blessed in our ability to be of service to others. Please do not lose the spirit of service in the teaching profession, as that will put you quickly on the path of asshole yoga teacher status. If you stay authentic and keep your teaching as an offering versus a perseveration of what you are getting in return, you will not devalue your service to others in a major way.

I am often blown away when students thank me after class and tell me that the practice has helped them overcome loss, pain, or difficulty. Yet all I am ever really trying to do is offer the space to grow, the place to have the yoga practice reveal itself. Any other gain that I make as part of the yoga business is secondary.

Think outside the Box

The industry standard for teacher pay per class in the United States can range anywhere from $20 to $50 per class. Not bad when you think that some master's-level professionals (including my husband), who have upward of $100,000 in student debt for that degree, don't even surpass $40 as an hourly rate in their fields. A yoga certificate that costs an average of $2,500 can demand that rate per class. In fact, a recent study showed that college graduates (ages twenty-one to twenty-four) are making an average hourly wage of $16.81 per hour, which equals a yearly salary of roughly $35,000. A new yoga teacher earning $25 per class doesn't sound so bad when you have a reality check like those statistics.

To sustain a living in the yoga teaching profession, however, most full-time yoga teachers need to teach at least three (sometimes more) classes per day, have a few private or corporate clients, and a few workshop rotations in the mix.

Many yoga teachers complain about what they get paid to teach, with the assumption that the studio owners are rolling in dough. There is a lot of deception around how much a studio is making per class when you look at a head count of attendance. It is quite common that a studio makes zero dollars a day in sales, yet still has to pay the teachers for the classes regardless. Then there is the overhead of rent, utilities (for a hot yoga studio, the winter heating bills can be as high as $900 a month per location), website costs, marketing programs like Facebook ads and Yelp, Internet service, federal and state taxes (you think you have a high tax bill?), necessary studio props, cleaning supplies, towel or laundry service, and so forth. During the slower seasons—summer, for example—a studio is lucky to break even at the end of the month. Ethical yoga studio owners are paying you before they are paying themselves.

In the era of yoga that exists today, a yoga class can cost anywhere from ten to twenty-eight dollars per class. You would be shocked to know, however, how many people prefer to pay for yoga at a highly discounted rate via outside promotions like Groupon and Classpass. This all must be taken into account when a studio determines the pay scale for teachers. I acknowledge that the system is flawed, with yoga teachers often having little to no medical benefits, no unpaid days off, no maternity leave, and independent contracts that require them to handle their own taxes at the end of the year, to name just a few of the stressors. Yet when I hear teachers complain, I often bite my tongue before saying that they chose to quit their jobs to teach full-time and often without the necessary due diligence.

This is the current business of teaching yoga. Twenty years ago, teachers taught for supplemental income, doing something that they loved while earning a little extra cash and a free studio membership. Nowadays, there are more and more full-time yoga teachers who are disgruntled that the grass is not necessarily greener on the other side.

As a yoga teacher, you must be creative in making the profession lucrative. Workshops can be very profitable if you have a topic of interest to share with the yoga community. If you have the opportunity to develop a unique workshop, it allows the students to dive a bit deeper than they can in an open class. Figure out an area of the practice that you feel passionate about and be the expert in your community. You can also make even more profit if the workshop can be repeated multiple times in a given time frame. The rates for workshops can be anywhere from 50 percent to 70 percent of gross profits, so that can be a great way to add additional income and expanded offerings into your teaching repertoire.

Be mindful, though: if you offer a workshop at one studio, then offer the same workshop at a different studio two blocks down the street, you are really just cutting into your own profits/attendance. Studios like to have unique offerings, but when the same event is offered in the immediate surroundings, it lessens the "unique" factor considerably. This can be enough to make a studio owner pass on offering your event or workshop.

Another way to include higher-profit offerings is to teach a series, with a specific beginning and end date. Studio owners and teachers love this because the clients commit to that given time frame in advance. Many studios offer series for fundamentals or "beginners." But you can get super creative with the type of series to offer. The sky is truly the limit; know your market and put yourself and your ideas out there! Some suggestions that I have seen market great interest are a yoga series for runners, restorative yoga, yoga for men, yoga for brides, yoga for teens, kids' yoga, 'tween yoga, chair yoga, senior yoga, inversion or arm balance, music-themed yoga…The list can go on and on. I have a yoga teacher friend who has combined her love of essential oils into a successful yoga and oil workshop. I have seen yoga and Thai massage events, yoga and acupuncture, and the like. Link up with other health-and-wellness professionals who have a specialty area and work in collaboration to create a unique experience for the students. Or seek additional training that will expand the depth and variety of your offerings.

In terms of teaching yoga, you really can have a fun, lucrative, and positive career. In fact, CNN posted in 2015 that the yoga-teaching profession is on the path of "great growth, great pay, and is a satisfying career." It does require thinking outside the box, however. You can generate additional income in the yoga business through corporate yoga contracts, private clients, or even teaching yoga courses at your local university.

With the tremendous popularity of social media, you can offer online classes, podcasts, and online tutorials. Teachers' yoga Instagram postings oftentimes speak louder than their true yoga résumés but can lead toward endorsements, traveling workshops, free yoga clothes, ambassadorships, and more. Yet, many practitioners find that the true essence of yoga gets distorted through such social media, lacking, in many cases, the philosophy behind the practice. The yoga profession is only as rewarding as you make it, so again, think outside the box and eventually realize there is no box.

Let's Dig deeper

Pose associated with Aparigraha: Pasasana (Noose Pose)

From Mountain Pose, bend your knees and lower your hips to your heels. Rotate your torso to the left and bring your upper right arm to the outside of your left leg, with your hands in a prayer position, at the heart. Option to use the Ganesha Mudra as an arm variation. Inhale to lengthen your spine and exhale to twist deeper, wringing out that which you do not need and being grateful for what you have. Repeat on the right side.

Mudra associated with Aparigraha: Ganesha Mudra

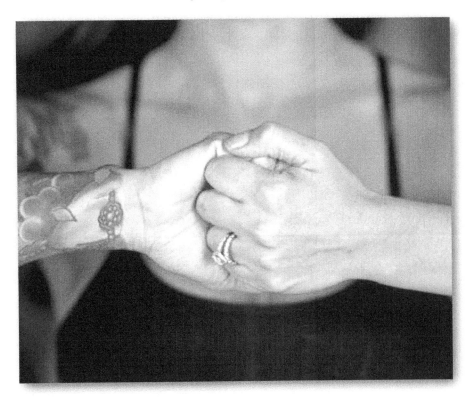

Ganesha Mudra is named after the Hindu deity who removes obstacles, but also puts obstacles in our way so we can realize our own strength and capabilities. To create this mudra, swivel the hands so that the fingertips point toward opposite elbows, with your right palm facing your heart. Bend the fingers and slide the hands away from each other until the fingers lock.

Mantra: *Om gam ganapatayei namaha*

With each exhale, invoke Ganesha (gam or ganapatayei) and his powers by chanting his name: *Om gam ganapatayei namaha*. (Om is the sound of the universe, and namaha means "name.")

What do you want? What is the value of this desire? Is it worth it?

Freedom of expression
time
relaxation
travel
rewarding career
lucrative pay

Does your desire have a greater value to the world?

What are you prepared to do about this desire?

Yes
train/teach

CHAPTER 7

Saucha

Saucha, or living purely, involves maintaining a cleanliness in body, mind, and environment so that we can experience ourselves in a higher resolution.

—Donna Farhi

The purification of the mind is very necessary.

—Swami Satchidananda

It is through your body that you realize you are a spark of divinity.

—B. K. S. Iyengar

Saucha brings us to the second limb of yoga, Niyama. The Niyamas have a more inward focus that outlines personal conduct intended to help us cultivate inner peace and equanimity. Niyama constitutes a code for living in a way that fosters a more yogic lifestyle through the choices we make. These practices extend the ethics provided by the Yamas to the yogi's internal environment of mind, body, and spirit. Niyama suggests that impurities in our external environment can both adversely affect our state of mind and prevent the attainment of spiritual wisdom.

The practices of Asana, Pranayama, and meditation cleanse and purify the body and mind and strengthen their capacity to maintain a pure state of being. We must therefore be conscious of what we take into our bodies and into our consciousness. This includes not only the foods we eat, but also the shows we watch on television and the people and places we surround ourselves with. We must assess how our habits, thoughts, and environment either diminish or contribute to the purity of our whole self.

Don't Be Dirty

In terms of cleanliness, this one is a no-brainer. Wear clean clothes, take a shower daily, or, at an utter minimum, wash your hands and feet before and after you teach. Yes, yogis are often all natural and earthy, but our odor should not be a distraction to those around us.

A teacher who had a great practice and students who really seemed to enjoy his classes once worked at our studio. One summer, he came to teach after spending a sunny day outside in the park, practicing Asana, Acro, tree climbing, and any other movement modality you can do in the outdoors. While I am sure it was a fulfilling and pleasant day for him, he came to the studio with a horrid body odor as well as grass particles still all over his clothes. Needless to say, a few yogis left and/or complained about the stench. Don't be an asshole; don't be dirty when you teach, assist, or interact with the students in your classes. We are encouraging full, deep breaths in this practice, and foul body odor should not hinder this.

A recent study conducted by New York University suggested that 80 percent of diseases are caught by direct or indirect contact, either by interacting with a person who is carrying germs or by touching a surface where those organisms are living. Unfortunately, both types of contact occur at high rates in yoga studios.

Students contracting germs and infections can permanently turn them off to the yoga practice. Think itchy skin bumps and rashes. Yuck!

Some facts about germs: Bacteria can survive anywhere from several hours to several days on inanimate objects, while viruses can linger on for weeks. Warm, humid conditions such as those found in Vinyasa, hot yoga, Mysore practice, or really any yoga class taught on a hot summer day can be a breeding ground for germs. Literally thousands of germs can linger in a group yoga setting. Just walking across an unsanitary studio floor is enough for a yogini to catch athlete's foot, plantar warts, or ringworm—or worse, Staphylococcus (MRSA), which has spread in frequency since the 1990s, perhaps with the influx of yoga centers and fitness facilities.

Yoga studios are not like restaurants, which are regulated and overseen by health departments. Even large gyms are overseen by sports club associations. At this time, yoga studios aren't subject to strict sanitary standards. Many have suffered from bedbugs, water contamination, and an influx of germs. This is why, as a yoga teacher, you can play a part in working together with the yoga community by taking the initiative for maintaining studio cleanliness. I am not suggesting cleaning toilets or even mopping floors (unless, of course, those are part of your designated duties as a teacher). If you see something that looks like it can use a wipe down after the class you taught, however, then please take the initiative to do so. Saucha. If you see the class has gotten pretty sweaty, remind students to wipe down their blocks and mats if the studio is equipped with a sanitizing station. Inform the studio owner when something needs maintenance or attention. We all benefit from cleanliness in our practice and in our teaching. After all, you are likely going to be walking around barefoot more than the students are.

Cleanse Your Thoughts

Purifying the mind is an intention of Saucha. During the course of the day, most of us experience a constant, random inner dialogue, with many repetitive, negative, and just downright unnecessary thoughts. When our senses are pulled in a variety of directions, our attention and energy moves in this haphazard way, too. This creates the mind chatter or "monkey mind" that the yoga practice aims to dissipate. Meditation and concentration are scientifically proven methods that bring random and haphazard mental activity under control. There are many mindfulness meditation practices that are beneficial not only to decrease mind chatter, but also to bring greater clarity to your thoughts, a reduction of anxiety, and an overall increase in happiness. Meditation, or *dhyana*, is a critical part of the Eight-Limbed Path of Yoga and should not be set on the sidelines behind yoga Asana. It should be intertwined with it.

Although we can consider yoga asana a moving meditation, or "meditation in motion," as Baron Baptiste calls it, there is no doubt that a grounded opportunity for stillness has great merit in the path of yoga and yoga teaching. I recommend that you take a few minutes per day to be still, to focus on breathing and eliminating the extra thoughts in your head. I also recommend offering this time to your students, as they may not have the awareness to do so without your guidance. Time for stillness doesn't have to be a huge chunk of your class; maybe offer just two minutes in the beginning as they get centered and grounded. Think of this as an offering to decrease the negative karmas that may have been accumulated by asshole-like actions of the past. I like to use this time in my classes to also quiet my own mind as I prepare to conduct the class with a greater state of presence. In doing so, I find that I can more easily see the goodness in all beings.

Let's Dig Deeper

Pose associated with Sauca: Viparita Karani (Legs-Up-the-Wall Pose)

Lie down on your back and extend your legs directly above your hips. This simple inversion facilitates the drainage of the lymphatic system. This drainage aids in purifying the body and boosting immunity. Rest your arms alongside your body with the palms turned up in preparation for the associated mudra.

Mudra associated with Sauca: Tattva Mudra

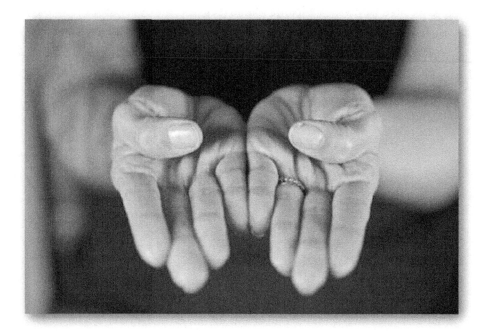

Bring each thumb to the base of the ring finger in Tattva Mudra. This hand gesture reminds us that the true nature of the Self, or our fundamental essence, is perfect, unchanging and pure.

Mantra: Om aim hridayam namaha

Chanting the heart mantra Om aim hridayam namaha (hridaya means "spiritual heart" or "heart center") ignites the heart fire to burn through whatever blocks us from recognizing our true Self.

Describe at least 5 ways that you can cleanse areas of your life, beyond just physical cleansing. What changes could you imagine this cleansing could bring about?

Nutrition - less meat, less sugar + weight loss health

Hydration - improved practice

Meditation - quiet mind

Communication - deeper friendships

more movement - mind cleaning

less TV -
more time for other things
more stillness + peace

CHAPTER 8

Santosha

CONTENTMENT

At the end of the day, what matters most is santosha: deep, abiding, everlasting contentment.

—Sumukhi

It isn't what you have or who you are or where you are or what you are doing that makes you happy or unhappy. It is what you think about it."

—Dale Carnegie

The result of contentment is total happiness.

—T. K. V Desikachar

Santosha is the second Niyamas of Patanjali's Eight-Limbed Path of Yoga. Santosha is about mastering the art of feeling at ease and at peace with yourself. It is often translated as "contentment," as this Niyamas lead us toward a more positive relationship with ourselves. This is so crucial because we cannot form authentic and sustainable relationships with our students until the connection with ourselves is intact and strong.

Even if you are dedicated in your yoga practice, there may still be that over-zealous thought of, "I'd be happier if..." going through your mind. Whether it's losing weight, teaching more, rocking a handstand, meeting the love of your life—regardless of what it is, you may feel there's something out there in the universe that can make you happier or more content. Don't get me wrong: pushing yourself toward a goal is not necessarily a bad thing, but it can be if you base your entire sense of worth or happiness upon it. Santosha is more about accepting where you are and being OK with that—then using that acceptance as a catapult to move forward.

Yoga teaches us that when we are perfectly content with all that life gives us, we are in position to attain true joy. Practicing contentment frees us from the unnecessary suffering of always wanting things to be different and instead fills us with gratitude and joy for all of our blessings.

Attitude of Gratitude

Be just as content when two people show up to your class as when one hundred fifty people show up. We should teach with as much vigor and passion every time we step into our space, regardless of class size or capability. Have an attitude of gratitude always. Use a smaller class size as a wonderful opportunity to fine-tune your teaching with informed individualized attention. Trust that the students who are meant to be in your class on any given day have found you. There are no mistakes; the universe is never wrong. The number of students does not define the teacher; however, the lack of ego and the generosity of your teaching do.

There is a yoga teacher who is based out of New York City. In the past few years, he has found much success in the yoga business with an innovative yoga prop that he designed. But before his notoriety on a larger scale, he was invited to come to Philadelphia as a guest teacher for a workshop at our studio. About a week before the event, he contacted me to see how many people were signed up. At the time, twelve had committed to attending.

His response was, "That's it?" and he proceeded to express his discontent and dissatisfaction with that class attendance. Needless to say, we canceled the workshop because it was clear that he did not find the trip to Philly worthwhile for that number of people. Of course, I, as well as the twelve people who signed up, were disappointed that he didn't honor the commitment, nor did he exhibit a sense of contentment or gratitude for those souls who wanted to be there. Even though it is likely that he could pack the studio now with his success, I do not even consider inviting him back.

This is just a reminder that you should not use the students as a channel to nourish yourself with affirmation and yoga teacher self-worth. Give generously, regardless of who shows up. Remember that we are teachers of not just Asana, but more importantly, Yama and Niyama.

Feel Good about Your Teaching

It is so easy to beat ourselves up after we teach a class that we feel could have been better. Our internal dialogue will rant, "Why didn't I hold pigeon longer...I cued my sun salutations too slow...I should have put reverse warrior before parsvokona-sana...Shit, I forgot a *whole sequence*." The negative mind chatter can go on and on.

It is those moments of awareness and introspection, however, that can bring us the most profound growth. It is those opportunities that help us shape our teaching for the next time we are given the opportunity.

It is likely that your class wasn't nearly as bad as you may have thought; after all, aren't we our own worst critics? Students are having their own experience on the mat, and often they don't even notice the little intricacies of our classes that we do as teachers.

If you make a mistake, take it lightly, Acknowledge the mishap to foster connection with the students. After all, even yoga teachers are still human. Make such acknowledgments with a swift lightheartedness that does not violate the student's trust in you, however. I say "swift" because you should not harp on the mishap; acknowledge it and move on. An apology is OK if done with confidence. If you are constantly apologizing with a nervous "Sorry, sorry, sorry," it is likely you will lose the class's ability to have faith in your words and guidance. Again, the likelihood that students even notice the aspects of the class you would have liked to do differently is slim. Too many repetitions of "sorry" only draw attention to them. If you do happen to forget a whole sequence, remember that a longer shavasana is never a bad thing.

A great tool to increase positive self-talk is to try talking to yourself the way you would actually talk to someone that you love. Wow, how about that?

Let's Dig Deeper

Pose associated with Santosha: Setu Bandha Sarvangasana (Supported Bridge Pose)

From a supine position, bend your knees and place your feet on the floor directly under them. Lift your hips and allow feelings of ease, contentment, and gratitude to wash over you in this heart-opening backbend. Place your arms by your sides, with the palms turned up in preparation of Jnana Mudra.

Mudra associated with Santosha : Jnana Mudra

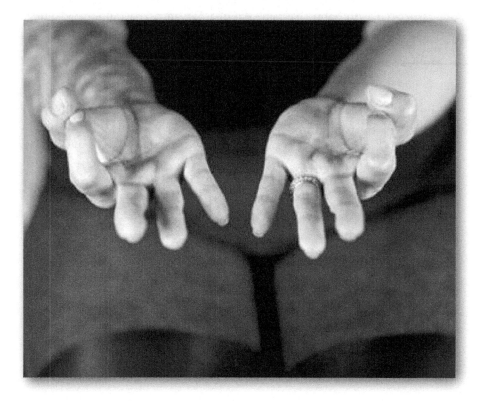

Tuck the tip of each index finger underneath the thumbs in a gesture of wisdom-Jnana Mudra.

Mantra: *Om shanti shanti shanti*

As you chant the mantra for peace (shanti), *Om shanti shanti shanti,* remember the wisdom and calmness that exists from peace and equanimity.

I feel happiest in my own skin when...

I am surrounded by people who love me & I enjoy being with.

Achieving Goals

Running a few miles

finishing an OTH/Pilates class Challenging

learning something new

leading others

CHAPTER 9

Tapas

DISCIPLINE

Life without Tapas is like a Heart without love.

—B. K. S Iyengar

Mere philosophy will not satisfy us. We cannot reach the goal by mere words alone. Without practice, nothing can be achieved.

—Swami Satchidananda

Genuine Tapas makes us shine like the sun...Then we can be a source of warmth and strength for others.

—George Feuerstein

Tapas is a yogic practice of intense self-discipline. Most simply, tapas is heat, specifically the kind of heat generated by yogic practices like yoga Asana and Pranayama. In the early scriptures, which still shape most of the yoga practiced today, *Tapas* refers to burning off impurities in the body. Perhaps more importantly tapas burns away the impurities in our thoughts and actions, bringing a more conscious awareness of our behaviors and interactions.

Tapas is also in effect anytime we are doing something that we don't want to do yet will have a positive effect on our lives. You can relate this to waking up early to practice, even though your mind may tell you to hit the snooze button or taking a class after a long day, despite the urge to go home and binge watch a show on Netflix. Tapas builds the willpower and personal strength necessary to become more dedicated to the practice of yoga. I also firmly believe that Tapas is required of an effective yoga teacher.

The Struggle Is Real

There is no doubt in my mind that there is a correlation to being a great teacher and the maintenance of a personal practice. Oftentimes when new teachers start teaching, they are so overly enthusiastic about sharing their passion that they fill all their available time with teaching. Although there is great merit in wanting to share and connect as much as possible with students, it is a sure way to burn *yourself* out, instead of burning out the impurities of the mind and body, as Tapas intends.

You must make time for your own practice. Having a consistent practice isn't the only requirement of being a good teacher, but it is definitely high on the list. You must continue to be a student, be open to learning, and be open to experiencing different teachers and different styles of yoga. There is always something to take with you from maintaining a practice, whether it be a cue that resonated with you or a sequence that felt amazing. Or it can be the opposite, noticing what you didn't like and being sure to learn from that, as well. Again, there is always something to be learned through your own personal practice. The discipline of tapas gives us the strategies necessary to be the most effective teachers we can be.

Your struggle as a yoga teacher to maintain your own practice is very real. You may have to get really creative with ways to fit the practice in. That is where true tapas comes into play. Start by simplifying your life in order to maintain the momentum in your own practice. Breathe a bit deeper, declutter your mind, and rid yourself of all that does not serve you. You may notice then that you have more time than you originally thought. I often suggest practicing yoga as soon as you wake up, first thing in the morning. If yoga is a priority in your life, then treat it as such. Use that time to separate from all other distractions, like checking your phone or your e-mail or even before drinking a breakfast smoothie. Separate from anything that puts the practice in a secondary position. The more we pile on before the practice, the more likely the practice time will just slip away. If you need to wake up an hour earlier to get your practice done, then set the alarm for that time and go to bed earlier to accommodate. Making time and space for yoga takes it out of the "should" mind-set and places it in the "must" mind-set. I have great admiration for an Ashtanga yoga teacher friend that starts her teaching at 5:45 a.m. each day. To compensate, however, she wakes up daily at 2:30 a.m. to fit in her own practice before she teaches. That is tapas if I have ever seen it.

In terms of the yoga practice itself, being extremely focused and disciplined does not mean perfecting the most advanced poses. Many times, yoga teachers feel the need to "master" what they consider to be difficult poses. With this mentality, the ego becomes attached to being "more advanced." With tapas, you need to identify ego-free goals that you fundamentally believe in. Let your goal be simple: to maintain a daily yoga practice. Remember, the more advanced poses will come, but they should not be the motivation. What matters most are the lessons to be learned along the way, the lessons that the practice unfolds for you.

Let's Dig Deeper

Pose associated with Tapas: Forearm Plank

Move into Sphinx pose propped up on your forearms with your toes curled under. On an exhalation, peel your body off the ground by pressing your forearms firmly into the earth. Press back through your heels to activate your legs. Draw your navel toward your spine and pull your shoulder blades away your ears and away from one another to avoid collapsing in the chest.

Mudra associated with Tapas: Mudra: Garuda Mudra

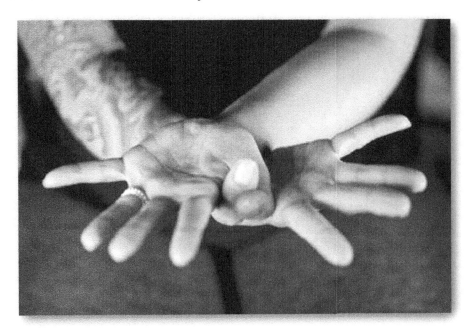

The perseverance that it takes to sustain forearm plank can inspire you to cultivate discipline and commitment. Turn your hands so that the palms face up and cross your right hand over your left, clasping your thumbs for Garuda Mudra, named after the eagle that Vishnu, the lord of preservation, rides.

Mantra: *Om agnaye namaha*

Summon that which you wish to transform through discipline, heat or fire by chanting the mantra *Om agnaye namaha*.

How do you know when you are trying too hard? What signals does your body send to you? Do you pay attention or ignore these signals?

Breathing changes

Heart Beats fast

Sense tension / overwhelmed feeling

What life accomplishments are most important to you? Identify the discipline that was or will be necessary to achieve such accomplishments.

HS Grad

Under Grad diploma

Birth/Raising of Kids

marriage to Scott

master's degree

1 of career

promos

CPRE

OHy TT

One year sober 2021

CHAPTER 10

Svadhyaya

SELF-STUDY

Knowing Yourself is the beginning of all wisdom.

—Aristotle

The peace of God is with them whose mind and soul are in
harmony, who are free from desire and wrath, who know
their own soul.

—Bhagavad Gita

Yoga is for internal cleansing, not external exercising.
Yoga means true self-knowledge.

—Pattabhi Jois

S vadhyaya is the ability to see our true divine nature through the contemplation of our life's lessons. To translate *svadhyaya* as "self-study" is rather precise. The first part of the word—*sva*—means "self." The second part—*dhyaya*—is derived from the verb root *dhyai*, which means "to contemplate, to think on, to recollect, or to call to mind." Thus, it works to translate *dhyaya* as "study"—to study one's own self.

Life presents endless opportunities to learn about ourselves; our flaws and shortcomings give us opportunities to grow and evolve, while our mistakes and ignorance allow us to learn. When we contemplate our actions, we can see our conscious and unconscious thoughts and desires more visibly.

In the West, we often equate self-study with therapy or psychoanalysis. This is not what was intended in yoga scripture, however. The analysis of our feelings, thoughts, and fantasies is not Svadhyaya. Rather, Svadhyaya suggests that any sacred or inspirational text that offers insight into the human condition can serve as a reflection, revealing our true nature back to us. Classical texts of this sort might include the Bible, Yoga Sutra, the Bhagavad Gita, the Talmud—generally, writings of any spiritual tradition that foster the path of deeper self-knowledge can encourage Svadhyaya.

In fact, Svadhyaya can refer to *any* activity that offers inspiration. This can include learning from a teacher, reciting hymns or mantras, creating a vision board, or listening to a sermon. In Svadhyaya, spiritual and/or inspiring teachings are tools to help us better understand ourselves. Through that understanding, we can change our attitudes and behavior more positively.

Always a Student

Similar to what we spoke of with Tapas, continue being a student. When you stop your desire to learn, you have become a bad teacher. You're not finished learning once you've graduated from a two-hundred-hour training program. Great teachers never stop studying and never stop being students. Be voracious in your reading of books that inspire you. Read books that not only stimulate you but also motivate you. Try to create links between your life on and off the mat so you can share your realizations with your students. Be the conduit for *their* self-study.

Seek out additional ways to learn and build in your teaching repertoire, whether in workshops, immersions, or additional teacher trainings. I sometimes joke that getting a two-hundred-hour yoga certification is like getting a bachelor's degree in yoga—but it merely scratches the surface of the vastness of this topic. I encourage you to go forward and get a yoga master's degree. Consistent learning will invigorate and inspire your teaching, giving you an ever-growing teaching toolbox to work from. It will also open you up to increased teaching opportunities and workshop specialties that can create a more lucrative yoga business. And, of course, never forget—practice, practice, practice.

Let's Dig Deeper

Pose associated with Svadhyaya: Padmasana (Lotus Pose)

Come to a comfortable seated pose with the tops of the feet resting on opposite thighs. As a modification, sit on a block, blanket, or bolster for additional support, or take Sukasana, or easy seat.

Mudra associated with Svadhyaya: Dhyana Mudra

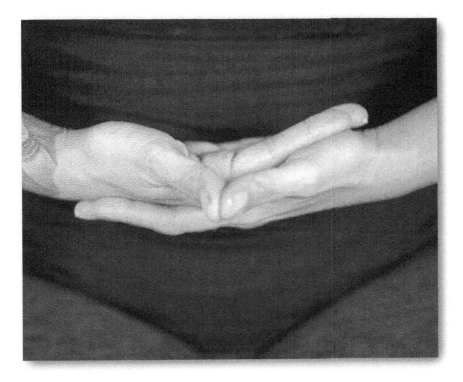

Bring your hands to the contemplative gesture of Dhyana Mudra by resting them, upturned, around the area of your navel with the right hand on top. Bring the thumbs together to touch at the tips, forming a triangle.

Mantra: *Tat tvam asi*

Gaze at the triangle while chanting *Tat tvam asi*, which can be translated as "You are what you seek." This mudra and mantra allow you to observe, without judgment, the desires, thoughts, cravings, and repetitive behaviors that cause you to disconnect from your True Self. This mantra is said to illuminate our dark shadows and sets us free from self-judgment.

Make a list of at least 20 things that inspire you. You can include books, quotes, paintings, people, websites, stores, etc.

Books

Artwork

People

music

CHAPTER 11

Ishvara Pranidhana

Surrender to the Lord

Surrender to what is. Let go of what was. Have faith in
what will be.

—Sonia Rocotti

Let us all dedicate our lives for the sake of the entire hu-
manity. With every minute, every breath, every atom of our
bodies we should repeat this mantra: "dedication, dedication, giving, giving, loving, loving."

—Swami Satchidananda

What would happen if you let everything to be exactly as
it is?

—Adyashanti

The term *Ishvara Pranidhana* is made up of two words: *Ishvara*, which
translates as "supreme being," "god," or "true self" and *Pranidhana*, which
means "fixing." In most translations of this Niyama, we're advised to

"surrender" to this supreme being or higher self. In a nutshell, this means to cultivate a deep and powerful relationship with the universe while making each action an offering to something bigger than us. Some studios find that discussing the concept of a god (or as in the Hindu tradition, many gods!) uncomfortable or even inappropriate in an open yoga class. Therefore, Ishvara Pranidhana can also be translated as "bowing" or acknowledging something grander than us. This interpretation can relate to many things, such as the source of life within and around us or the simple recognition that a higher consciousness exists.

In our Western culture, feelings of separateness and disconnection are so prevalent; just think of the 2016 election. There are many people who pride themselves on their strength and ability to dominate others. Our egos are too often the prevailing force in our actions and our goals. Ishvara Pranidhana represents surrender. This surrender does not mean weakness, however, and should not be looked upon negatively. In yoga the essence of surrender is far from the idea of defeat. Rather, we are surrendering our limited views of who we are by letting go of false identifications such as our gender, our career, our ethnicity, or our socioeconomic status. Once we let go of these false identifications, we can then create the space needed to feel the true nature of self, which is of limitless joy. When we let go of our false identifications, we can more readily see that we are all the same.

To practice Ishvara Pranidhana, we must have trust, self-discipline, and devotion. Although this can seem like an overwhelming task, the benefits are so powerful. Imagine trading in a grain of sand and receiving the entire universe in return. That is Ishvara Pranidhana.

Invite the Spiritual

There are a slew of new yoga studios in existence, with large studio corporations creating new styles of yoga, some that even pride themselves on stripping away the spiritual aspects of yoga to create a mere workout. In a sense, they are watering down all that yoga has to offer; however, I encourage you to celebrate the spiritual aspects of this practice with your students. This includes finding the words that help tap into your innate understanding of oneness and the presence of divinity. You may begin to see that this magic will make students keep coming to your classes.

If all you offer in your teaching is the mind-set of getting a thin yoga body and a handstand, then you will be offering only a surface level of yoga to your students. Yes, it is true that offering a yoga practice for merely the health benefits *will* result in practitioners feeling better, having more energy, and improving overall health. But this is not the depth the practice can and should allow. In order to really get the deepest benefit from the practice, you have to offer an intention on the spiritual journey of yoga. Trust that the reasons people practice yoga is beyond the physical benefits. I think that all humans on the planet can admit that they would like to be more peaceful, patient, and happy. All the necessary lessons that lead to that result will become evident within the yoga practice.

The reality of life is that shit happens. We are conditioned to avoid pain and attach to pleasure. There is always going to be something thrown in your way to disturb your peace, like traffic, bills, or a broken appliance, to name just a few things that can ruffle your feathers.

Think about water. We don't know the water's strength until a dam is put in its way. Only with that obstacle can the water reveal its true strength. Yoga is not about getting rid of all of our challenging experiences, nor is it a desire to take control of our external environment. In fact, it is quite the opposite. Yoga is about keeping your peace of mind regardless of whether you experience ease and joy or stress and pain. Attempting to change your external situations is a battle sure to be lost. Instead, teach your students that learning to gain control of their *thoughts* and *reactions* are skills way more worth mastering than a handstand. Teach that obstacles and challenges are simply put in our paths so our truest strength can emerge. Strive to take your students to this deeper level in your teaching. You will be playing an integral role in making the world a more peaceful place.

There are many ways you can invite and engage the spiritual aspects of yoga into a class, and the term "god" doesn't have to be mentioned at all. In fact, a simple chant of "om" is enough to embrace the divine. In fact, the word *om* represents *everything*. It is said to be the seed of all of creation. This seemingly small word contains all the power of the universe. It is the beginning, the middle, and the end—the past, present, and future. Om has vast popularity simply because of its vibration, felt not only within the room when chanted but also in the vibration it creates in the body. The sound is known to soothe the nervous system almost immediately. It has the ability to remove us from our mind chatter and prepares us to be more receptive and contemplative. In a class setting, it really does unite the group and create a sense of togetherness and community. Chanting a unified om aligns the body, mind, and spirit of the practitioners to become more as one. It is a grounding and peaceful sound that may be enough to set a spiritual tone to your classes.

Another way you can cultivate the willingness for your students to surrender is by encouraging the practice to be an offering; reiterate that this practice is about far more than just the by-products of a firm butt and lean muscles. Dedicating or offering all the effort on the mat brings the practitioners' own personal interpretation of Ishvara, or God, into their mind's eye. Remind the students to put aside criticisms and judgments and let go of the ego.

Consider theming your classes to include a deeper layer of the yoga practice, beyond just the physical. I highly recommend using references from traditional yoga teachings as part of your class inspiration. Perhaps in your teacher training, you read the Yoga Sutras and/or the Bhagavad Gita as part of the coursework. If you didn't, run to the bookstore now and pick up these books. They are timeless and so full of valuable knowledge. Every time you open one of those books, you can find something new to learn and share. That is the magic of a spiritual text. Although the yoga teachings are old, they are still applicable in contemporary times. In fact, they are hidden treasures of wisdom that can explain the human condition even in the present day.

Speak authentically by sharing your personal realizations and understandings of a sutra or philosophical concept, as this makes it real for your students. When you share, you are offering a bit of yourself to the class. During a child's pose, you can ask students rhetorical questions or suggest ways of thinking about yoga philosophy that allow students to examine their own feelings, thoughts, and experiences. It is a great way not only to invite the spiritual into your classes, but also to cultivate a relationship beyond just the poses. It makes yoga seem more like a way of life. Sometimes the yoga practice is enough to speak for itself. The divine can exist in the silence you allow between your cues or in the peace and quiet you perpetuate in the stillness of Shavasana.

Let's Dig Deeper

Pose associated with Ishvara Pranidhana: Pranamasana (Prayer Pose)

Lie on your belly, rest your forehead or chin on the ground and extend your arms out in front of you.

Mudra associated with Ishvara Pranidhana: Anjali Mudra

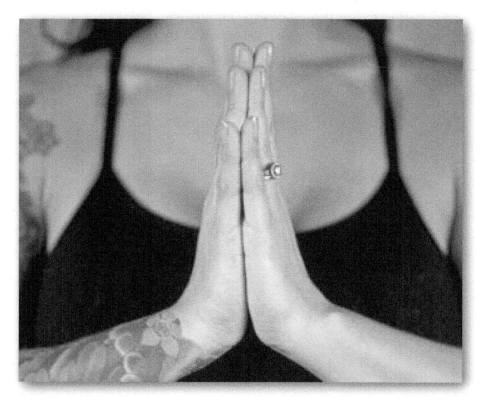

Bring your palms together at the heart center in Anjali Mudra. This gesture represents love and devotion.

Mantra: *Om*

Softly chant the sound of the universe-*Om*. Use this mantra as a way to surrender your fears, anxieties, and doubts. This will make life not only easier, but more joyful. Whether you offer the fruits of your practice to another, or bow to a force that is greater than yourself, the yoga practice teaches us that we actually contain the divine source of life within us. Ishvara Pranidhana reminds us that which we seek is already present within us.

What elements of your yoga practice have helped you to grow into your highest potential? What particular yoga pose(s) have taken you to that highest potential? How can you instill this to your students?

_____

_____

_____

_____

_____

_____

_____

_____

_____

_____

_____

_____

_____

_____

_____

_____

_____

_____

_____

_____

_____

_____

_____

_____

_____

_____

_____

_____

_____

Just remember, it all starts with you. Practice Yama and Niyama. Teach Yama and Niyama. Live and teach the practice of yoga fully and authentically. Don't be an asshole. Namaste.

About the Author

isa Mitchell (Ed.D, E-RYT 500) is a teacher at heart. Although always an advocate for yoga and well-being, she began her teaching career as a special-education teacher in the inner city of Philadelphia. She earned her doctorate degree in special education and researched the effects of the yoga practice and the ability for students with autism spectrum disorder to more freely initiate social interaction through the effects of yoga.

In 2007, Lisa and her husband, Dorian Mitchell, opened their first yoga studio, Dana Hot Yoga, in Bala Cynwyd, PA. Dana Hot Yoga currently has three locations throughout the surrounding Philadelphia area, where Lisa and Dorian presently teach. Lisa is a pioneering force in the Dana Hot Yoga Teacher-Training Program, and she leads yoga retreats both locally and internationally. She has been a contributing writer for Mindbodygreen.com and was cast on *Yoga Sutra Now* on the Veria Network. Lisa is also a mom of three children, a cat, and an English bulldog.

Made in the USA
Monee, IL
30 March 2021

64157080R10085